COOKBOOK AND MEAL PLAN FOR RECENTLY DIAGNOSED DIABETES

Nourishing Recipes and Practical Guidance for **Type 2 Diabetes** Management

Tara Wason

CONTENTS

1

Introduction

Type 2 diabetes, a chronic condition characterized by insulin resistance and elevated blood sugar levels, has emerged as a significant health concern globally. This introduction delves into the intricate web of factors contributing to its rise and emphasizes the pivotal role of proper nutrition in managing and preventing this condition.

Overview of Type 2 Diabetes

In recent decades, the prevalence of Type 2 diabetes has surged, creating a pressing need for comprehensive understanding and effective management strategies. Type 2 diabetes is fundamentally rooted in insulin resistance, where the body's cells fail to respond adequately to insulin, leading to an accumulation of glucose in the bloodstream. This metabolic disorder can result in a range of complications, including cardiovascular issues, kidney disease, and nerve damage.

Exploring the causes and risk factors unveils a complex interplay of genetic predisposition, lifestyle choices, and environmental influences. Genetics may lay the groundwork, but lifestyle factors such as sedentary behaviour, unhealthy dietary habits, and obesity often trigger the onset of Type 2 diabetes. Unravelling this intricate tapestry provides a foundation for developing tailored interventions that encompass both prevention and management.

Importance of Proper Nutrition

Amidst the multifaceted landscape of Type 2 diabetes, the role of proper nutrition emerges as a cornerstone in promoting overall health and mitigating the impact of the condition. Nutrition serves as a powerful tool in managing blood sugar levels, enhancing insulin sensitivity, and averting complications associated with diabetes.

The journey towards optimal nutrition involves understanding the significance of balanced meals, nutrient-dense foods, and mindful eating. Crafting a diet that prioritizes whole grains, lean proteins, fruits, and vegetables not only aids in controlling blood glucose but also contributes to weight management—a critical aspect in Type 2 diabetes care.

Furthermore, the influence of dietary patterns on the body's inflammatory response and oxidative stress underscores the need for an anti-inflammatory and antioxidant-rich diet.

Exploring the nuances of the glycaemic index and glycaemic load becomes imperative, as it guides individuals towards selecting foods that have a minimal impact on blood sugar levels.

As I delve into the importance of nutrition, it becomes evident that dietary choices extend beyond the immediate goal of managing diabetes. They play a crucial role in preventing the progression of the condition, reducing the risk of associated complications, and fostering overall well-being.

In this comprehensive exploration, I embark on a journey through the intricacies of Type 2 diabetes, recognizing nutrition as a powerful ally in the pursuit of health. By unravelling the layers of this condition and understanding the symbiotic relationship between lifestyle and well-being, we lay the groundwork for a nuanced and informed approach to Type 2 diabetes management.

2

Understanding Diabetes

Type 2 diabetes, a complex metabolic disorder, demands an in-depth exploration to grasp its intricacies fully. This section delves into the basics of Type 2 diabetes, its profound effects on the body, and the essential lifestyle adjustments required for effective management.

Basics of Type 2 Diabetes

To gain a deeper insight into the fundamentals of Type 2 diabetes, it's essential to grasp the intricate dynamics involving insulin, glucose, and the body's regulatory mechanisms. Insulin, a key hormone produced by the pancreas, plays a crucial role in facilitating the absorption of glucose by cells for energy. In individuals with Type 2 diabetes, however, cells develop resistance to insulin, hindering an effective response.

This resistance initiates a domino effect. As cells resist insulin's signals to take in glucose, the pancreas responds by producing more insulin. Over time, this constant demand places strain on the pancreas, leading to diminished insulin production. The dual challenge of insulin resistance and reduced insulin secretion results in elevated blood sugar levels.

Understanding the intricacies of glucose metabolism is paramount. Carbohydrates, the primary source of glucose, undergo digestion, releasing sugars into the bloodstream. In a well-regulated system, insulin facilitates the absorption of this glucose by cells. In Type 2 diabetes, this process malfunctions, causing an accumulation of glucose in the blood—a condition termed hyperglycaemia.

Examining the role of the liver introduces another layer of complexity. Normally responsible for storing and releasing glucose as needed, the liver may malfunction in individuals with Type 2 diabetes. Instead of maintaining a balanced glucose level, the liver may release excess glucose into the bloodstream, exacerbating hyperglycaemia.

Furthermore, understanding impaired beta-cell function sheds light on the progressive nature of Type 2 diabetes. As these cells, responsible for insulin production, face continuous stress, their ability to generate insulin diminishes, complicating the body's efforts to regulate blood sugar effectively.

In summary, the basics of Type 2 diabetes revolve around a disruption in the intricate interplay of insulin, glucose, and cellular response. This disruption not only impacts immediate blood sugar levels but also sets the stage for long-term complications, emphasizing the need for a holistic and proactive approach to diabetes management.

Comprehending these fundamentals serves as a solid foundation for individuals diagnosed with Type 2 diabetes. Armed with this knowledge, they can engage in informed conversations with healthcare providers, make educated decisions about treatment options, and actively participate in managing their health.

Effects on the Body

To delve further into the impact of Type 2 diabetes on the body, it's crucial to uncover the intricate physiological changes that occur, affecting diverse organ systems and contributing to a range of complications.

1. Cardiovascular Ramifications:

The cardiovascular system shoulders a significant burden in the context of Type 2 diabetes. Prolonged hyperglycaemia accelerates the development of atherosclerosis, resulting in the narrowing and hardening of arteries. This sets the stage for complications like hypertension, coronary artery disease, and an elevated risk of heart attacks and strokes. The interplay between heightened glucose levels and oxidative stress contributes to endothelial dysfunction, further compromising cardiovascular health.

2. Renal Issues:

The kidneys, essential for maintaining fluid and electrolyte balance, undergo increased stress in uncontrolled diabetes. Diabetic nephropathy, a progressive kidney disease, may ensue, marked by impaired kidney function and heightened albuminuria. Recognizing the intricate link between hyperglycaemia and renal complications underscores the significance of meticulous diabetes management to prevent lasting kidney damage.

3. Neurological Ramifications:

Type 2 diabetes exerts a profound influence on the nervous system, resulting in diverse neurological complications. Peripheral neuropathy, characterized by tingling, numbness, and pain in the extremities, is a prevalent outcome. Additionally, diabetes correlates with a heightened risk of cognitive impairment and conditions like Alzheimer's disease. These neurological consequences highlight the necessity for a comprehensive diabetes care approach that extends beyond mere blood sugar control.

4. Ocular Complications:

The eyes are not immune to the impact of Type 2 diabetes. Diabetic retinopathy, a condition characterized by damage to the blood vessels in the retina, emerges as a significant concern. If left unmanaged, it can lead to impaired vision and blindness. Regular eye examinations and vigilant blood sugar control are essential in preventing and managing diabetic retinopathy.

5. Influence on Wound Healing:

Type 2 diabetes can hinder the body's ability to heal wounds efficiently. Elevated blood sugar levels can result in compromised circulation and weakened immune function, causing delays in the healing process. Individuals with diabetes face an increased risk of infections and experience sluggish wound healing, particularly in the extremities.

Understanding these multifaceted impacts on the body underscores the urgency of adopting a holistic approach to Type 2 diabetes management. Beyond controlling blood sugar levels, interventions must address cardiovascular risk factors, kidney health, neurological well-being, ocular health, and wound care. Proactive measures, including regular medical check-ups and lifestyle adjustments, become imperative in mitigating diabetes's impact on diverse organ systems and enhancing overall quality of life.

Lifestyle Adjustments

In navigating the landscape of Type 2 diabetes management, recognizing the central role of lifestyle adjustments becomes pivotal. These adaptations encompass changes in dietary patterns, consistent physical activity, stress mitigation, and holistic well-being practices, offering a comprehensive strategy that extends beyond pharmaceutical interventions.

1. Dietary Changes:

Understanding the intricacies of Type 2 diabetes involves a thoughtful examination of dietary choices. Moving beyond traditional carbohydrate counting, adopting a well-rounded, nutrient-rich diet is essential. Managing portion sizes, practicing mindful eating, and incorporating a diverse range of whole foods are key elements. The focus on selecting foods with a low glycaemic index supports stable blood sugar levels, promoting sustained energy and minimizing post-meal spikes.

2. Regular Exercise:

Physical activity emerges as a potent ally in the management of Type 2 diabetes. Customizing exercise routines based on individual preferences and abilities not only aids in weight control but also enhances insulin sensitivity. Engaging in a combination of aerobic exercises and strength training contributes to overall health, fostering cardiovascular well-being and reducing the risk of diabetes-related complications.

3. Stress Alleviation:

Recognizing the intricate link between stress and blood sugar levels underscores the significance of stress management in diabetes care. Integrating stress-reducing practices such as mindfulness, meditation, and deep breathing techniques can have profound effects on both mental and physical health. Actively addressing stress contributes to improved blood sugar regulation and enhances overall quality of life.

4. Quality Sleep:

The role of sufficient sleep-in diabetes management should not be underestimated. Sleep deprivation can disrupt insulin sensitivity and glucose metabolism, exacerbating the challenges faced by individuals with Type 2 diabetes. Prioritizing healthy sleep habits and establishing consistent sleep patterns contribute to enhanced metabolic health.

5. Regular Monitoring and Health Check-ups:

Vigilant monitoring of blood sugar levels, coupled with routine medical check-ups, constitutes a fundamental aspect of effective diabetes management. This proactive approach facilitates timely adjustments to treatment plans, ensuring interventions align with the evolving health needs of individuals. Regular health assessments also aid in identifying potential complications early on, enabling prompt intervention and prevention.

6. Community Involvement and Support:

The journey of managing Type 2 diabetes is often made more manageable through community engagement and support. Participating in diabetes support networks, whether in-person or online, provides a platform for individuals to exchange experiences, gather insights, and find encouragement. Building a supportive network enhances resilience and cultivates a sense of community that positively impacts mental well-being.

In essence, lifestyle adjustments in Type 2 diabetes management embrace a holistic framework that extends beyond pharmaceutical solutions. By adopting dietary modifications, incorporating regular physical activity, managing stress, prioritizing adequate sleep, and fostering connections within a supportive community, individuals can empower themselves to proactively address their health. These adjustments not only contribute to improved blood sugar control but also enhance overall well-being, paving the way for a healthier and more fulfilling life despite the challenges posed by Type 2 diabetes.

3

Meal Planning Fundamentals

Meal planning is a cornerstone in the effective management of Type 2 diabetes, providing a structured approach to nourishment that aligns with specific health needs. This section delves into the fundamental aspects of meal planning, emphasizing the nutritional requirements for individuals with diabetes, the importance of portion control, and the art of choosing the right foods to maintain optimal blood sugar levels.

Nutritional Requirements for Diabetics

Exploring the nutritional needs of individuals with Type 2 diabetes involves a nuanced examination of macronutrients—carbohydrates, proteins, and fats—and their impact on blood sugar management.

1. Carbohydrates:

Quality Takes Precedence: Prioritizing the quality of carbohydrates is crucial. Opting for whole grains, legumes, and vegetables not only provides essential nutrients and fibre but also aids in blood sugar control and overall satisfaction.

Mindful Glycaemic Index Choices: Considering the glycaemic index (GI) of foods assists in selecting carbohydrates that have a gradual impact on blood sugar levels. Choosing low-GI options, such as quinoa and sweet potatoes, ensures sustained energy without causing abrupt spikes.

2. Proteins:

Lean Protein Emphasis: Emphasizing lean protein sources is fundamental. Choices like poultry, fish, tofu, and legumes offer essential amino acids without excessive saturated fats. Distributing protein intake evenly throughout the day promotes lasting energy and balanced macronutrient consumption.

Balanced Protein Distribution: Spreading protein intake across meals contributes to sustained energy and satiety, preventing excessive snacking and maintaining a well-rounded nutritional profile.

3. Fats:

Promoting Healthy Fats: The inclusion of healthy fats is vital for those with Type 2 diabetes. Avocados, nuts, seeds, and olive oil provide monounsaturated and polyunsaturated fats, supporting heart health and overall well-being. Monitoring the intake of saturated and trans fats is essential to mitigate cardiovascular risks.

Limiting Saturated and Trans Fats: Keeping a check on saturated and trans fats is critical. Foods high in these fats, such as processed snacks and certain animal products, can contribute to insulin resistance and negatively impact lipid profiles.

4. Fibre:

Fibre's Essential Role: Incorporating dietary fibre is a key consideration. Found in fruits, vegetables, whole grains, and legumes, fibre aids digestion and helps manage blood sugar levels.

It also contributes to a feeling of fullness, supporting effective weight management.

Hydration and Fibre: Ensuring adequate water intake, especially with increased fibre consumption, promotes digestive health and minimizes potential gastrointestinal discomfort associated with a high-fibre diet.

5. Micronutrients:

Vitamins and Minerals Focus: Ensuring sufficient intake of vitamins and minerals is crucial. Foods rich in potassium, magnesium, and vitamin D, such as leafy greens, nuts, seeds, and fatty fish, support overall health and may offer specific benefits for individuals with diabetes.

Sodium Monitoring: Considering the link between diabetes and cardiovascular risk, monitoring sodium intake is essential. Limiting processed and high-sodium foods contributes to maintaining optimal blood pressure levels.

Understanding these nutritional intricacies empowers individuals with Type 2 diabetes to make informed dietary decisions. Tailoring their nutritional intake based on these guidelines not only aids in blood sugar control but also addresses broader health considerations, fostering a proactive approach to overall well-being.

Portion Control

Diving deeper into the concept of portion control unveils a nuanced strategy that goes beyond mere quantity, encompassing mindful eating habits, a balanced distribution of macronutrients, and the significance of consistent meal timing.

1. Grasping Portion Sizes:

Visualizing Adequate Servings: Developing a clear understanding of appropriate portion sizes involves visualizing standard servings for various food groups. Tools like measuring cups, visual guides, or everyday objects can assist in accurately gauging portion sizes.

Progressive Awareness: Over time, individuals can train themselves to better estimate portions, cultivating a more intuitive and adaptable approach to portion control. This skill becomes particularly valuable in social settings where precise measurements may not be feasible.

2. Equilibrium in Macronutrients:

Crafting Well-Balanced Meals: Portion control is not solely about volume; it includes the distribution of macronutrients—carbohydrates, proteins, and fats. Achieving a harmonious balance ensures that meals contribute to sustained energy, satiety, and stable blood sugar levels.

Utilizing the Diabetes Plate Method: A practical approach to portion control, the diabetes plate method involves visually dividing a plate into segments for various food groups. This method facilitates a proportional intake of carbohydrates, proteins, and non-starchy vegetables, simplifying meal planning for those with Type 2 diabetes.

3. Meal Timing and Frequency:

Consistent Meal Spacing: Distributing meals throughout the day fosters more stable blood sugar levels. Incorporating nutritious snacks between meals helps prevent extended periods of hunger and avoids overeating during main meals. A regular meal schedule contributes to enhanced glycaemic control.

Synchronizing with Medication: Considering the timing of meals concerning medication is pivotal. Aligning meals with medication schedules optimizes treatment plan efficacy and prevents blood sugar fluctuations. Maintaining consistency in meal timing establishes a routine that supports overall metabolic health.

4. Mindful Eating Techniques:

Enjoying Each Bite Mindfully: Mindful eating entails relishing each bite and being attuned to flavours, textures, and the overall eating experience. This practice not only enhances meal enjoyment but also cultivates heightened awareness of hunger and fullness cues.

Minimizing Distractions: Reducing distractions during meals, such as watching TV or using electronic devices, fosters a mindful eating atmosphere. Being present and engaged with the act of eating encourages better recognition of satiety, preventing excessive consumption.

5. Hydration's Role in Portion Control:

Water's Contribution to Fullness: Adequate hydration contributes to feelings of fullness, aiding in portion control. Drinking water before meals can help manage appetite, curbing excessive calorie intake. Additionally, staying well-hydrated supports overall health and metabolic function.

Grasping and implementing these elements of portion control empowers individuals with Type 2 diabetes to effectively manage their food intake. It's not merely about limiting quantity; it's about fostering a mindful and intuitive connection with food. These strategies contribute not only to glycaemic control but also to overall well-being, promoting a sustainable and health-conscious approach to eating.

Expanding this exploration into the realm of selecting the appropriate foods involves a comprehensive examination of the qualities defining a healthful diet for those managing Type 2 diabetes. This entails giving priority to whole foods, balancing macronutrients, considering glycaemic index, and making informed choices for overall well-being.

1. Prioritizing Whole Foods:

Choosing Nutrient-Dense Options: The cornerstone of selecting the right foods involves prioritizing whole, nutrient-dense choices. Opting for fruits, vegetables, whole grains, lean proteins, and healthy fats ensures a diverse array of essential vitamins, minerals, and fibre crucial for overall health.

Minimizing Processed Food Intake: Steering away from highly processed and refined foods is essential. These often contain added sugars, unhealthy fats, and elevated sodium levels, all of which can exacerbate blood sugar fluctuations and contribute to other health issues.

2. Achieving Macronutrient Balance:

Diversifying Protein Selections: Making wise protein choices involves incorporating diversity. Including lean sources like poultry, fish, legumes, and tofu not only provides essential amino acids but also supports stable blood sugar levels.

Optimizing Healthy Fat Choices: Opting for healthy fats from sources like avocados, nuts, seeds, and olive oil contributes to heart health. Striking a balance between monounsaturated and polyunsaturated fats while limiting saturated and trans fats is crucial for diabetes management.

3. Practicing Mindful Eating:

Appreciating Flavours and Textures: Mindful eating goes beyond the selection of foods to how they are enjoyed. Savouring flavours and textures, being fully present during meals, and paying attention to satiety cues foster a positive and mindful relationship with food.

Reducing Distractions: Minimizing distractions during meals enables individuals to concentrate on the act of eating, decreasing the likelihood of overconsumption and encouraging a more mindful approach to nourishment.

4. Considering Glycaemic Index:

Preferring Low-Glycaemic Options: Utilizing the glycaemic index (GI) guides the selection of carbohydrates that have a gradual impact on blood sugar levels. Opting for low-GI foods like whole grains, legumes, and non-starchy vegetables effectively manages post-meal glucose levels.

Balancing Carbohydrates: Striking a balance between carbohydrates, proteins, and fats within each meal supports overall glycaemic control. This approach ensures sustained energy and prevents drastic blood sugar fluctuations.

5. Hydration and Nutrient Intake:

Water as the Primary Choice: Prioritizing water as the primary beverage is vital. It hydrates without contributing extra calories or sugars.

Limiting sugary drinks, including sodas and fruit juices, supports hydration while avoiding unnecessary spikes in blood sugar.

Incorporating Herbal Teas and Infusions: Adding herbal teas and infusions to the diet provides a flavourful and healthful alternative. These beverages offer hydration while delivering antioxidants and other beneficial compounds.

6. Tailored Meal Planning:

Adapting Choices to Personal Preferences: Acknowledging individual tastes and cultural considerations is crucial. Customizing meal plans based on personal preferences ensures sustained adherence to a healthful diet.

Consulting Healthcare Professionals: Seeking advice from healthcare professionals, such as dietitians and nutritionists, facilitates personalized and evidence-based dietary recommendations. This collaborative approach ensures that dietary choices align with specific health objectives.

In essence, choosing the right foods for individuals with Type 2 diabetes involves a holistic strategy encompassing whole foods, balanced macronutrients, mindful eating practices, considerations of glycaemic index, and personalized meal planning. This comprehensive approach not only supports glycaemic control but also fosters overall well-being, offering a

guideline for sustainable health management.

4

Diabetic-Friendly Recipes

Embarking on a journey to create diabetic-friendly recipes involves a thoughtful selection of ingredients, consideration of portion sizes, and attention to nutritional balance. This section will explore a variety of recipes tailored for individuals managing Type 2 diabetes, focusing on breakfast options, lunch and dinner recipes, and snack ideas.

Breakfast Options

Crafting a varied and satisfying breakfast menu for individuals handling Type 2 diabetes involves integrating an assortment of nutrient-dense elements to foster sustained energy and blood sugar management.

1) Quinoa and Berry Breakfast Bowl:

Ingredients:

❖ Quinoa

❖ Assorted berries (strawberries, blueberries, raspberries)

❖ Chopped nuts (almonds, walnuts)

❖ Greek yoghurt

Instructions:

- ❖ Prepare quinoa following package directions.

- ❖ Combine cooked quinoa with an array of fresh berries in a bowl.

- ❖ Garnish with a scoop of Greek yogurt and sprinkle chopped nuts for added texture and wholesome fats.

Benefits:

- ❖ Quinoa supplies complex carbohydrates and protein.

- ❖ Berries introduce natural sweetness and antioxidants.

- ❖ Nuts contribute healthy fats and extra protein.

2) Vegetable Omelette with Whole Grain Toast:

Ingredients:

- ❖ Eggs

- ❖ Mixed veggies (bell peppers, spinach, tomatoes)

- ❖ Olive oil

❖ Whole grain bread

Instructions:

❖ Beat eggs and sauté mixed veggies in

olive oil until tender.

❖ Pour beaten eggs over vegetables to create

an omelette.

❖ Serve with a slice of toasted whole grain

bread.

Benefits:

❖ Eggs offer high-quality protein.

❖ Vegetables provide fibre and essential nutrients.

❖ Whole grain toast contributes complex carbohydrates and additional fibre.

3) Greek Yogurt Parfait:

Ingredients:

❖ Greek yogurt

❖ Mixed berries

❖ Granola (low-sugar)

Instructions:

- ❖ Layer Greek yogurt with sliced berries and a small amount of granola in a glass or bowl.

- ❖ Repeat layers according to preference.

Benefits:

- ❖ bring natural sweetness and antioxidants.

- ❖ Greek yogurt serves as a rich source of protein.

❖ Berries Granola offers a crunchy texture

and extra fibre.

4) Spinach and Feta Egg Muffins:

Ingredients:

❖ Eggs

❖ Fresh spinach

❖ Feta cheese

❖ Cherry tomatoes

Instructions:

- ❖ Whisk eggs and incorporate fresh spinach, crumbled feta, and diced cherry tomatoes.

- ❖ Pour the mixture into muffin tins and bake until set.

Benefits:

- ❖ Eggs supply protein and vital nutrients.

- ❖ Spinach contributes fibre and essential vitamins.

❖ Feta adds savoury flavour without excessive saturated fat.

These breakfast selections cater to diverse palates while integrating vital nutrients. They are formulated to deliver a mix of carbohydrates, proteins, and fats, ensuring a gratifying and health-conscious beginning to the day for those managing Type 2 diabetes.

Lunch and Dinner Recipes

Developing fulfilling and nutritious lunch and dinner choices for those managing Type 2 diabetes involves a meticulous selection of components, emphasizing lean proteins, whole grains, and a variety of vegetables to promote overall health and blood sugar regulation.

1) Grilled Salmon with Quinoa and Roasted Vegetables:

Ingredients:

❖ Salmon fillet

❖ Quinoa

❖ Mixed vegetables (broccoli, carrots, bell peppers)

Instructions:

- ❖ Grill salmon with a light coating of olive oil until it easily flakes.

- ❖ Prepare quinoa following package instructions.

- ❖ Roast an assortment of vegetables and serve them over quinoa alongside grilled salmon.

Benefits:

- ❖ Salmon contributes omega-3 fatty acids for heart health.

❖ Quinoa delivers complex carbohydrates

and protein.

❖ Vegetables provide fibre, vitamins, and

minerals.

2) Turkey and Vegetable Stir-Fry:

Ingredients:

❖ Lean ground turkey

❖ Assorted vegetables (bell peppers, broccoli, snap peas)

❖ Low-sodium soy sauce

Instructions:

❖ Brown ground turkey in a pan.

❖ Incorporate a mix of vibrant vegetables

and stir-fry until they're tender.

❖ Finish with a drizzle of low-sodium soy

sauce and serve over brown rice or

cauliflower rice.

Benefits:

❖ Turkey serves as a lean protein source.

❖ Vegetables supply fibre and essential nutrients.

❖ Soy sauce enhances flavour without excessive sodium.

3) Mediterranean Chickpea Salad:

Ingredients:

❖ Chickpeas (canned or cooked)

❖ Cherry tomatoes

❖ Cucumber

❖ Feta cheese

❖ Olive oil and lemon dressing

Instructions:

❖ Combine chickpeas, cherry tomatoes, diced cucumber, and crumbled feta in a bowl.

❖ Drizzle with olive oil and lemon dressing.

❖ Toss gently and serve as a refreshing
salad.

Benefits:

❖ Chickpeas supply protein and fibre.

❖ Tomatoes and cucumbers add vitamins
and antioxidants.

❖ Feta provides a savoury element.

**4) Grilled Chicken and Vegetable
Skewers:**

Ingredients:

- ❖ Chicken breast, cubed

- ❖ Bell peppers, cherry tomatoes, red onions

- ❖ Olive oil and herb marinade

Instructions:

- ❖ Marinate chicken in a blend of olive oil and herbs.

- ❖ Thread chicken cubes, bell peppers, cherry tomatoes, and red onions onto skewers.

- ❖ Grill until chicken is fully cooked, and vegetables are tender.

Benefits:

- ❖ Chicken offers lean protein.

- ❖ Colourful vegetables supply vitamins and antioxidants.

- ❖ Olive oil marinade introduces healthy fats.

These lunch and dinner recipes prioritize a mix of macronutrients and vital nutrients while considering blood sugar levels. Adjusting portion sizes based on individual requirements and seeking guidance from healthcare professionals or dietitians ensures personalized dietary support.

Snack Ideas

Creating satisfying and diabetes-friendly snacks involves choosing options that balance macronutrients, control portion sizes, and provide sustained energy without causing significant blood sugar fluctuations. Here are additional snack ideas designed for individuals managing Type 2 diabetes:

1) Avocado and Whole Grain Crackers:

Ingredients:

❖ Avocado

❖ Whole grain crackers

Instructions:

❖ Mash ripe avocado and spread it on whole grain crackers.

❖ Sprinkle with a bit of salt and pepper for extra flavour.

Benefits:

❖ Avocado contributes healthy fats and

fibre.

❖ Whole grain crackers offer complex

carbohydrates and additional fiber.

2) Cottage Cheese with Berries:

Ingredients:

❖ Low-fat cottage cheese

❖ Mixed berries (strawberries, blueberries,

raspberries)

Instructions:

❖ Combine low-fat cottage cheese with a

handful of fresh berries.

❖ Drizzle with a touch of honey or add a

sprinkle of cinnamon for sweetness.

Benefits:

❖ Cottage cheese provides protein.

❖ Berries add natural sweetness, fibre, and

antioxidants.

3) Almond Butter and Apple Slices:

Ingredients:

❖ Unsweetened almond butter

❖ Apple slices

Instructions:

❖ Spread a thin layer of unsweetened almond butter on apple slices.

❖ Optionally, sprinkle with chia seeds or a dash of cinnamon.

Benefits:

❖ Almond butter offers healthy fats and

protein.

❖ Apples provide natural sweetness and

fiber.

4) Yogurt and Granola Parfait:

Ingredients:

❖ Unsweetened Greek yogurt

❖ Low-sugar granola

❖ Sliced banana or berries

Instructions:

❖ Layer unsweetened Greek yogurt with a small amount of low-sugar granola and fresh fruit slices.

❖ Repeat layers according to preference.

Benefits:

❖ Greek yogurt supplies protein.

❖ Low-sugar granola adds crunch and additional fibre.

5) Edamame Snack:

Ingredients:

*   Steamed edamame

*   Sea salt

Instructions:

*   Steam edamame and sprinkle with a pinch

    of sea salt.

*   Enjoy as a satisfying and protein-rich

    snack.

Benefits:

❖ Edamame provides plant-based protein.

❖ It's a convenient and portion-controlled

snack.

These snack ideas offer diverse flavours and textures while ensuring a balanced intake of macronutrients. Adapting portions to individual needs and seeking guidance from healthcare professionals or dietitians ensures personalized support for effective blood sugar management.

5

Weekly Meal Plans

Embarking on a journey to manage Type 2 diabetes involves not just individual meals but the orchestration of a well-rounded weekly meal plan. This section will guide you through the creation of sample meal plans tailored to different preferences and shed light on the significance of balancing nutrients across the week.

Sample Meal Plans for Different Preferences

Developing a range of meal plans that cater to diverse tastes ensures individuals managing Type 2 diabetes can relish a spectrum of flavours while adhering to healthy dietary practices. Let's further elaborate on sample meal plans tailored to different culinary preferences:

1. **Classic Mediterranean Delight:**

- **Monday:**

Breakfast: Spinach and feta omelet paired with whole grain toast.

Lunch: Grilled chicken Greek salad with a lemon vinaigrette.

Dinner: Mediterranean quinoa with baked cod and roasted vegetables.

- **Wednesday:**

Breakfast: Nutty yogurt parfait featuring mixed berries, honey, and assorted nuts.

Lunch: Hummus and whole grain pita served alongside lentil and vegetable soup.

Dinner: Greek-style salad accompanying eggplant and zucchini lasagna.

- **Friday:**

Breakfast: Smoked salmon and cream cheese on a whole grain bagel with capers.

Lunch: Falafel wrap with tahini dressing and a side of tabbouleh.

Dinner: Mediterranean-style shrimp pasta with whole wheat noodles.

2. Asian Fusion Harmony:

- **Tuesday:**

Breakfast: Brown rice congee paired with a soft-boiled egg and green onions.

Lunch: Teriyaki tofu stir-fry with broccoli and brown rice.

Dinner: Sushi-inspired bowl with quinoa, avocado, cucumber, and salmon.

- **Thursday:**

Breakfast: Matcha green tea smoothie infused with banana and chia seeds.

Lunch: Miso broth-infused ramen noodle bowl featuring vegetables and grilled chicken.

Dinner: Thai curry with beef and vegetables, served with cauliflower rice.

- **Saturday:**

Breakfast: Vietnamese-style iced coffee accompanied by whole grain toast and almond butter.

Lunch: Bibimbap bowl featuring marinated tofu, vegetables, and a fried egg.

Dinner: Steamed fish with ginger and soy sauce, served with jasmine rice and bok choy.

3. Hearty Plant-Based Indulgence:

- **Sunday:**

Breakfast: Vegan pancakes drizzled with maple syrup and adorned with mixed berries.

Lunch: Quinoa and black bean stuffed bell peppers, complemented by guacamole.

Dinner: Lentil and vegetable curry accompanied by brown rice.

- **Tuesday:**

Breakfast: Acai bowl topped with granola, coconut flakes, and fresh fruit.

Lunch: Chickpea and sweet potato Buddha bowl adorned with tahini dressing.

Dinner: Zucchini noodles paired with tomato and basil sauce, garnished with nutritional yeast.

- **Thursday:**

Breakfast: Chia seed pudding served with almond milk and sliced kiwi.

Lunch: Vegan burrito bowl featuring black beans, corn, avocado, and lime.

Dinner: Portobello mushroom burgers served with sweet potato wedges.

These diversified meal plans showcase the array of options available for those managing Type 2 diabetes. Customizing meals based on specific tastes not only enhances adherence to a healthful diet but also contributes to a positive and enjoyable culinary experience.

Balancing Nutrients Throughout the Week

Ensuring a comprehensive intake of nutrients throughout the week is crucial for effective blood sugar management and overall well-being. Let's explore in greater detail the strategies for maintaining equilibrium among key nutrients during the week:

Proteins:

Varied Sources: Include diverse lean proteins like poultry, fish, tofu, legumes, and dairy across different meals.

Uniform Distribution: Distribute protein consumption evenly throughout the week, ensuring each meal contains a quality protein source.

Carbohydrates:

Optimal Choices: Select complex carbohydrates such as whole grains, vegetables, and legumes to provide sustained energy.

Controlled Intake: Monitor carbohydrate consumption, spreading it consistently across the week to prevent blood sugar spikes.

Fats:

Healthy Selections: Choose healthy fats from sources like avocados, nuts, seeds, and olive oil.

Equitable Composition: Maintain a balance between saturated and unsaturated fats, integrating a mix of plant-based and animal-based fats.

Fibre:

Abundant Selections: Prioritize high-fibre foods like fruits, vegetables, whole grains, and legumes for digestive health.

Steady Consumption: Ensure a steady fibre intake throughout the week, promoting a sense of fullness and stable blood sugar levels.

Vitamins and Minerals:

Colourful Variety: Consume a range of colourful fruits and vegetables to access a spectrum of essential vitamins and minerals.

Rotational Strategy: Rotate through different vegetables and fruits weekly to diversify nutrient intake.

Hydration:

Adequate Water Intake: Stay well-hydrated by drinking water consistently throughout the day, reducing the risk of dehydration.

Smart Beverage Choices: Limit sugary drinks and opt for herbal teas or infused water to enhance flavour without added sugars.

Portion Management:

Conscious Eating: Practice mindful eating and control portions to prevent excessive intake and support weight management.

Smaller Servings: Use smaller plates and bowls as a natural way to regulate portion sizes.

Diversity and Moderation:

Versatile Menu: Integrate a variety of foods to ensure a comprehensive nutrient profile.

Moderate Indulgences: Enjoy occasional treats in moderation, offsetting them with nutrient-rich choices for overall dietary equilibrium.

Maintaining nutrient balance throughout the week involves purposeful planning and prudent decision-making. By incorporating a broad spectrum of nutrient-rich foods, individuals can not only effectively manage blood sugar levels but also foster overall vitality and well-being. This approach guarantees the body receives a diverse array of essential nutrients, promoting sustained health.

6

Managing Blood Sugar Levels

Effective management of blood sugar levels is a cornerstone for individuals navigating Type 2 diabetes. This section delves into key aspects, focusing on monitoring and testing, adjusting meal plans, and the vital role of physical activity in maintaining glycaemic control.

Monitoring and Testing

Effective oversight and examination play pivotal roles in the management of blood sugar levels, providing crucial insights that empower individuals to make informed decisions for their diabetes care.

- **Continuous Glucose Monitoring (CGM):**

Real-time Insights: CGM systems furnish an uninterrupted flow of real-time data on blood glucose levels.

Trend Analysis: Continuous monitoring enables users to observe trends and patterns, aiding in the identification of the impact of various factors on blood sugar.

Alerts and Notifications: Automated alerts can notify individuals of imminent high or low blood sugar levels, allowing proactive adjustments.

- **Self-Monitoring of Blood Glucose (SMBG):**

Day-to-Day Monitoring: Frequent testing with portable glucometers offers snapshots of blood sugar throughout the day.

Mealtime Adjustments: Pre-meal and post-meal readings assist in adjusting insulin doses or modifying meal plans based on individual responses.

Overnight Monitoring: Occasional overnight testing provides insights into nocturnal blood sugar patterns.

- **HbA1c Testing:**

Three-Month Average: HbA1c testing reflects average blood sugar levels over the past three months.

Long-Term Assessment: Provides a broader perspective on glycaemic control, aiding healthcare professionals and individuals in assessing the effectiveness of the overall diabetes management plan.

Treatment Adjustments: Changes in treatment plans may be recommended based on HbA1c results.

- **Interpreting Results:**

Target Ranges: Understanding individualized target blood sugar ranges guides decision-making.

Postprandial Monitoring: Evaluating blood sugar levels after meals offers insights into the impact of dietary choices.

Variability Assessment: Recognizing and addressing blood sugar variability contributes to more stable control.

Technology Integration:

Smartphone Applications: Many contemporary glucometers synchronize with smartphone apps, facilitating data tracking and analysis.

Data Sharing: Remote monitoring capabilities allow healthcare providers to assess real-time data and collaborate with individuals for personalized adjustments.

Integration with Insulin Pumps: Some CGM systems can communicate with insulin pumps to automate insulin delivery based on real-time readings.

- **Educational Support:**

Understanding Patterns: Education on interpreting blood sugar patterns empowers individuals to make timely adjustments.

Self-Management Training: Training programs guide individuals in effectively utilizing monitoring tools for optimal self-management.

Continuous Learning: Staying informed about advancements in monitoring technology and strategies ensures individuals are equipped with the latest tools and knowledge.

- **Psychosocial Impact:**

Emotional Well-being: Regular monitoring can have psychosocial implications, and it's essential to address emotional aspects.

Support Networks: Engaging with support groups or healthcare professionals can help individuals navigate the emotional challenges associated with continuous monitoring.

Positive Reinforcement: Celebrating successes, irrespective of size, reinforces a positive mindset in managing blood sugar levels.

Continuous enhancement in monitoring technologies and increased accessibility to testing tools empowers individuals to take an active role in their diabetes management. The integration of real-time data, education, and emotional support creates a holistic approach to monitoring that extends beyond numbers, focusing on overall well-being.

Modifying Meal Plans as Required

Customizing meal plans is a dynamic aspect of managing diabetes, demanding adaptability to evolving circumstances and individual responses. Let's explore further into strategies for adjusting meal plans as necessary to optimize blood sugar control.

- **Flexible Carbohydrate Management:**

Observing Glycaemic Response: Noting how diverse carbohydrates impact blood sugar aids in understanding individualized reactions.

Carbohydrate Counting Adaptability: Tailoring carbohydrate intake based on daily activities, stress levels, and overall health facilitates personalized glycaemic control.

Learning from Trends: Recognizing patterns in post-meal blood sugar readings helps refine carbohydrate choices.

- **Adaptability in Meal Timing:**

Aligning with Daily Routines: Adjusting meal times to synchronize with daily activities and energy needs promotes stable blood sugar levels.

Snack Adjustments: Strategically including snacks between meals prevents significant blood sugar fluctuations.

No Universal Schedule: Acknowledging that ideal meal timing varies among individuals, with experimentation being essential to finding the most effective routine.

- **Moderation in Protein and Fat Intake:**

Balancing Nutrients: Ensuring a blend of proteins, fats, and carbohydrates in each meal supports sustained energy release.

Portion Control: Monitoring portion sizes of proteins and fats prevents overconsumption and supports overall caloric equilibrium.

Diverse Protein Choices: Including a variety of protein sources, such as lean meats, fish, tofu, and legumes, diversifies nutrient intake.

- **Adjustments After Meals:**

Monitoring Postprandial Readings: Tracking blood sugar levels after meals provides immediate insights into the meal's impact.

Identifying Trigger Foods: Recognizing specific foods causing notable postprandial spikes allows for strategic modifications.

Gradual Changes: Implementing gradual adjustments avoids abrupt shifts that might disrupt overall glucose management.

- **Prioritizing Hydration and Fibre:**

Maintaining Hydration: Adequate water intake supports overall health and aids in digestion.

Focus on Fibre-Rich Foods: Emphasizing high-fibre choices like fruits, vegetables, and whole grains promotes satiety and stabilizes blood sugar.

Balanced Soluble and Insoluble Fibre: Ensuring a mix of soluble and insoluble fibre supports digestive health and glycaemic control.

- **Collaboration with Healthcare Professionals:**

Regular Consultations: Periodic discussions with healthcare providers empower individuals to make informed decisions regarding meal plan adjustments.

Guidance from Nutritionists: Seeking advice from nutritionists or dietitians ensures personalized meal plans align with health objectives.

Integration of Professional Feedback: Incorporating insights from healthcare professionals enhances the effectiveness of the overall diabetes management strategy.

- **Considering Cultural and Lifestyle Factors:**

Honouring Cultural Preferences: Acknowledging and incorporating dietary preferences based on culture fosters a sustainable approach to meal planning.

Sustainable Modifications: Implementing changes aligned with an individual's lifestyle ensures long-term adherence.

Promoting Enjoyable Eating: Prioritizing enjoyable meals contributes to overall well-being and encourages consistency in following adjusted meal plans.

Adjusting meal plans as necessary is a continual process that requires a blend of self-awareness, nutritional knowledge, and openness to adaptation. This personalized approach not only optimizes blood sugar control but also promotes a positive and enduring relationship with food.

Infusing Physical Activity

The inclusion of physical activity stands as a fundamental element in blood sugar management for those with diabetes. This section delves into various facets of infusing physical activity as a proactive strategy for enhancing overall well-being.

- **Tailored Exercise Regimens:**

Consulting with Experts: Crafting exercise plans in consultation with healthcare professionals and fitness specialists ensures personalized routines in line with health objectives.

Gradual Intensity Adjustments: Incrementally adapting exercise intensity and duration aligns with individual capabilities, promoting sustainable engagement.

Regular Evaluations: Consistent assessments allow for adjustments based on evolving fitness levels and health considerations.

- **Varied Exercise Approaches:**

Cardiovascular Activities: Participation in aerobic exercises like walking, jogging, or swimming boosts cardiovascular health and bolsters insulin sensitivity.

Strength Building: Including resistance exercises fosters muscle development, contributing to improved glucose control.

Flexibility and Balance Practices: Engaging in activities such as yoga or tai chi enhances overall well-being, supporting an active and balanced lifestyle.

- **Personalized Physical Activity Objectives:**

Realistic Goal Setting: Establishing achievable physical activity goals ensures sustained commitment and motivation.

Progress Tracking: Regularly monitoring and celebrating milestones creates positive reinforcement, encouraging ongoing dedication.

Adaptation to Preferences: Integrating activities that individuals enjoy heightens the likelihood of maintaining a consistent exercise routine.

- **Post-Exercise Nutrition:**

Strategic Timing: Consuming balanced post-exercise snacks prevents hypoglycaemia and aids in muscle recovery.

Protein and Carbohydrate Balance: Incorporating a mix of protein and carbohydrates in post-exercise nutrition supports effective recovery and stabilizes blood sugar levels.

Hydration Significance: Maintaining adequate post-exercise hydration is crucial for overall health and optimal metabolic function.

- **Monitoring Exercise Impact:**

Observing Blood Sugar Responses: Understanding how different exercise types and durations influence blood sugar levels allows for informed adjustments.

Recording Activity Patterns: Maintaining an exercise log facilitates the identification of trends, enabling individuals to correlate physical activity with blood sugar fluctuations.

Regular Assessments: Periodic reviews with healthcare professionals ensure alignment between the chosen exercise plan and overall diabetes management goals.

- **Social Backing and Group Engagements:**

Motivation from Community: Participating in physical activities with others provides motivation and a sense of community support.

Involvement of Family and Friends: Encouraging family and friends to join in physical activities fosters a supportive environment.

Group Classes or Clubs: Participation in exercise classes or clubs tailored for individuals with diabetes can offer camaraderie and shared experiences.

- **Mindful Movement Practices:**

Mind-Body Connection: Engaging in practices such as mindfulness-based activities or gentle movements enhances the connection between mind and body.

Stress Reduction: Incorporating activities focusing on relaxation and stress reduction contributes to overall well-being and may positively impact blood sugar levels.

Consistent Integration: Regular inclusion of mindful movement practices complements traditional exercise routines.

Safety Considerations:

Regular Check-ins with Healthcare Providers: Periodic consultations with healthcare professionals ensure alignment between chosen physical activities and overall health objectives.

Gradual Progression: Incremental adjustments in exercise intensity and duration prevent injuries and accommodate individual fitness levels.

Foot Care Awareness: Particularly crucial for individuals with diabetes, maintaining proper foot care minimizes the risk of complications related to neuropathy and circulation.

Infusing physical activity into daily life is a dynamic process that yields numerous advantages beyond blood sugar management. From personalized exercise plans to diverse activities and mindful practices, the inclusion of movement contributes to a comprehensive approach to diabetes care, promoting not only physical health but also mental and emotional well-being.

7

Tips for Dining Out

Dining out can be a delightful experience, but for individuals managing Type 2 diabetes, it often comes with the challenge of navigating menus to make healthy choices. Additionally, handling social situations while adhering to dietary needs requires a thoughtful approach. This section provides comprehensive guidance on making informed decisions at restaurants and managing social aspects of dining out.

Thoughtful Menu Exploration:

✔ Many contemporary menus dedicate specific sections to healthier alternatives. Explore these segments to discover dishes crafted with nutritional considerations.

✔ Pay close attention to how dishes are described. Terms like "grilled," "roasted," or "steamed" often signal healthier cooking methods in contrast to "fried" or "sauteed."

Accessing Allergen and Nutrition Details:

✔ If comprehensive nutrition information or

allergen details aren't readily available,

don't hesitate to request them. This

empowers you to make informed and

health-conscious choices.

✔ Some establishments provide nutritional

insights through their applications.

Consider utilizing these resources for a

comprehensive understanding of the menu.

Personalized Customization:

✔ Many restaurants are open to customizing dishes based on dietary preferences. Feel free to request modifications, such as swapping sides or adjusting seasoning, to align with your needs.

✔ Utilize customization options to assemble a well-rounded meal featuring lean proteins, whole grains, and an abundance of vegetables.

Beverage Considerations:

✔ Opt for water, unsweetened tea, or other

low-calorie drinks to avoid excessive

sugar intake.

✔ When choosing alcoholic beverages, opt

for lower-sugar options and be mindful of

portion sizes. Consider diluting wine with

water or selecting light beer.

Pre-Meal Planning:

✔ Consuming a small, nutritious snack

before heading to a restaurant can help

curb hunger, preventing impulsive and less healthy choices.

✔ Many restaurants publish their menus online. Previewing them in advance allows you to plan your selections and make informed decisions prior to arrival.

Embracing Diverse Cuisines:

✔ Global cuisines often offer a rich array of flavourful and nutritious choices. Explore cuisines like Mediterranean, Japanese, or Indian, which frequently feature dishes with an emphasis on vegetables, lean proteins, and healthy fats.

✔ Many international cuisines highlight grilled or steamed options, providing healthier alternatives to fried or heavily sauced dishes.

Appetizer as a Main Course:

Some appetizers can serve as satisfying main courses. Look for options that include protein and vegetables, such as grilled shrimp, vegetable skewers, or a protein-enhanced salad.

Sharing with Companions:

✔ Sharing multiple dishes with companions allows for a varied culinary experience without the need for large portions of any single dish.

✔ When dining with friends or family, encourage the selection of dishes aligned with your dietary objectives, fostering a supportive and health-conscious atmosphere.

Monitoring Hidden Sugars:

✔ Exercise caution with sauces and dressings that may contain hidden sugars. Even seemingly healthy salads can become high in sugar if dressed with sweet vinaigrettes or condiments.

✔ Opt for dishes with fresh, whole ingredients rather than heavily processed options, as the latter often harbour hidden sugars and undesirable additives.

Considering Side Dishes:

Pay attention to side dishes, as they can significantly contribute to overall calorie and carbohydrate content. Prioritize steamed vegetables, side salads, or whole grains.

Making health-conscious choices at restaurants involves a blend of menu awareness, careful planning, and effective communication. By embracing these guidelines, individuals managing Type 2 diabetes can navigate restaurant dining with assurance, striking a balance between enjoying flavourful meals and adhering to health objectives.

Acknowledging Social Influence:

✔ Recognize that social gatherings often

come with expectations and peer influence regarding food choices. Stay true to your health objectives while navigating these social dynamics.

✔ Take opportunities to inform those close

to you about your dietary requirements, promoting comprehension and encouragement in social settings.

Effective Verbal Expression:

✔ Communicate your dietary preferences and restrictions confidently and diplomatically. Clearly express your needs, enabling others to understand the significance of your dietary decisions.

✔ Encourage open conversations about your dietary needs, emphasizing that your well-being is a priority. This openness can contribute to a more supportive social atmosphere.

Influencing Venue Choices:

✔ When feasible, recommend restaurants or

locations offering a range of options

suitable for your dietary requirements.

This proactive approach sets a positive

tone for social occasions.

✔ Opt for venues accommodating diverse

dietary preferences, ensuring everyone

can enjoy a satisfying meal.

Pre-Event Discussions:

✔ If attending events with planned meals,

inform organizers about your dietary

needs beforehand. This allows for adjustments and minimizes potential discomfort.

✔ Discuss menu choices before arriving at a

restaurant. This proactive approach helps you make well-informed decisions and ensures suitable options are available.

Strategic Ordering:

✔ Select items strategically from the menu

that align with your health goals. This demonstrates your dedication to well-being without drawing unnecessary attention to your choices.

✔ Practice assertiveness when ordering to ensure your needs are met without causing discomfort. Tactful communication contributes to a positive dining experience.

Balancing Special Occasions:

✔ Acknowledge that special occasions may present tempting food options. Plan for moderation, balancing indulgence with mindful choices to maintain overall health.

✔ Consider incorporating physical activities into social occasions, such as a pre- or post-meal walk with companions.

Navigating Unfamiliar Cuisines:

✔ When dining at a place with unfamiliar cuisine, familiarize yourself with common dishes and their nutritional profiles beforehand. This knowledge assists in making informed choices.

✔ Don't hesitate to ask restaurant staff for advice on suitable options or modifications based on your dietary preferences.

Managing Buffet Challenges:

✔ Before serving yourself at a buffet, take a moment to survey the available dishes. This allows for mindful decision-making rather than succumbing to the appeal of all offerings.

✔ Opt for nutrient-dense options, focusing on salads, lean proteins, and vegetables, and limiting portions of high-calorie or sugary items.

Encouraging Supportive Discussions:

✔ Openly discuss your health goals with friends and family, encouraging conversations that support your journey. Positive reinforcement contributes to a supportive social circle.

✔ Shift the focus of social gatherings to non-food accomplishments or activities, reinforcing the idea that enjoyment and connection extend beyond meals.

Graceful Declines and Explanations:

✔ Politely decline offers of foods that don't align with your health goals. Express appreciation for the gesture while emphasizing your commitment to a specific dietary path.

✔ Seize opportunities to educate friends and family about your diabetes management. This can dispel misconceptions and foster empathy and understanding.

Staying Committed to Choices:

✔ During social occasions, remind yourself
of your health objectives and the
dedication you've made. This mental
reinforcement strengthens your resolve to
make informed choices.

✔ Acknowledge the triumphs of making
health-conscious choices in social
settings. Recognize your efforts and their
positive impact on your overall
well-being.

Creating a Support System:

✔ Surround yourself with individuals who comprehend and respect your dietary decisions. Building a supportive network can make social situations more comfortable and enjoyable.

✔ If feasible, engage with friends or support groups with similar health goals. Shared understanding fosters camaraderie in navigating social scenarios.

Gracefully handling social situations involves effective communication, thoughtful planning, and maintaining a positive outlook. By integrating these suggestions, individuals managing Type 2 diabetes can not only adhere to their dietary requirements but also cultivate supportive and understanding social environments.

8

Emotional Well-Being

Emotional well-being is a crucial aspect of managing Type 2 diabetes, encompassing coping mechanisms, support structures, and effective stress management strategies. In this section, we will explore how individuals can navigate the emotional dimensions of their health journey.

Coping with the Diagnosis

Reflective Journaling:

Maintaining a journal becomes an avenue for expressing emotions and thoughts regarding the diabetes diagnosis. Consistently reflecting on experiences and hurdles can bring clarity and serve as a cathartic outlet.

Expressing Creativity:

Engaging in creative pursuits, be it through art, writing, or music, provides a unique channel for emotional expression. Creative endeavours serve as therapeutic tools, enabling individuals to process emotions and find solace in self-expression.

Holistic Healing Approaches:

Some individuals find solace in exploring alternative therapies like acupuncture, massage, or herbal remedies. While not substitutes for medical care, these holistic approaches can complement conventional treatments and contribute to overall well-being.

Realistic Outlook:

Coping with a diabetes diagnosis is a journey, and it's crucial to set realistic expectations. Recognize that adapting to lifestyle changes and accepting emotions may take time, allowing for progression at a manageable pace.

Mindfulness for Stress Reduction:

Participation in formal mindfulness programs, such as Mindfulness-Based Stress Reduction (MBSR), equips individuals with practical tools to manage stress and navigate the emotional complexities linked with diabetes. MBSR emphasizes present-moment awareness and non-judgmental acceptance.

Positive Support Networks:

Cultivate relationships with individuals who offer positive encouragement and understanding. Sharing feelings with those providing support without judgment builds a network that reinforces emotional well-being.

Acknowledging Achievements:

Celebrate both minor and major achievements in diabetes management. Whether adopting a new healthy habit or achieving a specific health goal, acknowledging progress contributes to a sense of achievement and elevates morale.

Continuous Learning Opportunities:

Attend workshops or classes focused on diabetes management for continuous learning. Ongoing education not only deepens knowledge but also reinforces a proactive approach to understanding and addressing the condition.

Spiritual and Emotional Exploration:

For those inclined toward spirituality, seeking guidance from a spiritual leader or engaging in activities aligning with personal beliefs can offer solace and assist in coping with the emotional facets of a diabetes diagnosis.

Adaptive Coping Strategies:

Acknowledge that coping strategies may evolve over time. Remaining open to trying new methods and adapting coping techniques based on individual needs and changing circumstances is key.

Participation in Clinical Trials and Research:

Some individuals find purpose and empowerment in participating in clinical trials or research related to diabetes. Contributing to scientific advancements fosters a positive outlook and a connection to a broader community working towards improved solutions.

Engagement in Peer Mentoring Programs:

Participate in peer mentoring programs where individuals who have successfully coped with their diabetes diagnosis can offer guidance and support to those navigating similar challenges. Shared experiences create understanding and camaraderie.

Cultivation of Resilience:

Embrace resilience as a fundamental quality for navigating the emotional impact of a diabetes diagnosis. Resilience involves adapting to challenges, learning from setbacks, and maintaining a positive outlook despite difficulties.

Coping with a diabetes diagnosis involves a dynamic process that includes self-reflection, creative expression, and the development of supportive networks. By incorporating these varied coping strategies, individuals can confront the emotional aspects of their health journey with strength and a sense of empowerment.

Fostering Supportive Networks

Virtual Diabetes Communities:

Engaging in virtual diabetes communities provides a readily accessible and continuous source of assistance. These platforms offer a space for sharing experiences, seeking advice, and receiving real-time encouragement from individuals familiar with the intricacies of living with diabetes.

Therapeutic Counselling Services:

Seeking support from counsellors or therapists specializing in diabetes-related emotional struggles can be highly beneficial. These professionals offer a confidential space to explore feelings, develop coping mechanisms, and cultivate a resilient mindset.

Family Participation in Diabetes Education:

Actively involving family members in diabetes education sessions fosters a united front against the challenges of managing the condition. A well-informed family not only provides practical assistance but also offers emotional understanding and motivation.

Structured Diabetes Education Programs:

Participating in structured diabetes education programs that include group sessions cultivates a sense of camaraderie. Collaborating, learning together, and discussing challenges with peers can create a supportive environment.

Supportive Work Environment:

In the workplace, fostering an open and understanding environment is crucial. Communicating with supervisors and colleagues about specific needs related to diabetes management promotes a supportive atmosphere.

Regular Check-Ins with Healthcare Professionals:

Beyond medical consultations, regular check-ins with the broader diabetes care team, including dietitians and educators, reinforce ongoing support. Regular discussions allow for addressing the emotional aspects of diabetes management.

Tailored Mobile Apps for Diabetes:

Utilizing personalized mobile apps designed for diabetes management enhances self-care. These apps often include features for tracking progress, setting reminders, and accessing educational resources, providing continuous support.

Utilizing Telehealth Services:

Leveraging telehealth services ensures consistent access to healthcare professionals, even from a distance. Remote consultations facilitate ongoing discussions about emotional well-being and personalized approaches to managing diabetes.

Community Workshops and Events:

Attending workshops and events organized by local diabetes organizations or healthcare institutions offers opportunities to connect with others facing similar challenges. These gatherings provide a sense of community and shared learning.

Social Media Advocacy and Awareness:

Engaging in diabetes advocacy through social media platforms can create a broader network of support. By raising awareness and sharing personal experiences, individuals contribute to a supportive online community.

Establishing Diabetes Buddy Systems:

Forming personal diabetes buddy systems pairs individuals for mutual support. Sharing experiences, exchanging tips, and having a dedicated support partner create a more personalized and empathetic network.

Collaborative Exercise Groups:

Joining exercise groups specifically tailored for individuals with diabetes combines physical activity with social connection. These groups often serve as a dual platform for health improvement and emotional support.

Educational Resources for Loved Ones:

Providing educational materials to friends and family about diabetes fosters a deeper understanding. This, in turn, equips loved ones to offer informed and empathetic support on the emotional aspects of the diabetes journey.

Integration of Mental Health Screening:

Integrating routine mental health screenings into diabetes care ensures that emotional well-being remains a priority. Identifying and addressing emotional challenges early contributes to long-term mental health.

Creating a Diabetes Support Calendar:

Developing a diabetes support calendar outlines regular check-ins, educational sessions, and social activities related to diabetes management.

This structured plan provides a roadmap for ongoing support.

Empowering Self-Help Groups:

Facilitating self-help groups where peers take on leadership roles fosters a sense of empowerment. These groups can become a valuable source of emotional support, shared knowledge, and encouragement.

Building and nurturing a robust support system involves a multifaceted approach, incorporating professional, personal, and community-based resources. By leveraging these diverse avenues of support, individuals can navigate the challenges of diabetes with resilience and a sense of shared empowerment.

Programs for Mindfulness-Based Stress Reduction (MBSR):

Participation in programs that focus on Mindfulness-Based Stress Reduction (MBSR) offers an organized approach to managing stress. These programs typically incorporate guided mindfulness practices, meditation, and mindful movements, promoting heightened present-moment awareness and stress reduction.

Practices for Mindful Breathing:

Including mindful breathing exercises in daily routines acts as a pragmatic tool for reducing stress. Deliberate, deep breaths can activate the body's relaxation response, soothing the nervous system and fostering a sense of calm.

Engaging in Yoga and Tai Chi:

Regular participation in yoga or Tai Chi sessions combines physical activity with mindfulness. These practices emphasize controlled breathing, focused attention, and fluid movements, contributing to physical well-being and stress relief.

Biofeedback and Techniques for Relaxation:

Exploring biofeedback and relaxation techniques enables individuals to gain control over physiological responses to stress. Methods like progressive muscle relaxation or biofeedback devices provide real-time feedback, aiding in stress management.

Cognitive-Behavioural Therapy (CBT):

Cognitive-Behavioural Therapy (CBT) effectively identifies and modifies thought patterns that contribute to stress. By tackling negative thinking and implementing positive coping strategies, CBT empowers individuals to manage stress more effectively.

Therapeutic Arts Expression:

Participation in expressive arts therapy, including activities like art, music, or dance, offers a creative outlet for expressing and processing stress. These outlets serve as non-verbal forms of communication, promoting emotional well-being.

Maintaining Journals for Emotional Expression:

Regular journaling serves as an avenue for emotional expression and stress release. Writing about emotions, challenges, and positive experiences fosters self-awareness and facilitates emotional release.

Acupuncture and Pressure Point Techniques:

Exploring traditional approaches like acupuncture or acupressure can be beneficial for stress management. Rooted in Eastern medicine, these practices aim to balance the body's energy, promoting relaxation and stress reduction.

Nature Walks and Outdoor Pursuits:

Spending time in nature, whether through walks, hikes, or other outdoor activities, has proven benefits for stress reduction. Nature provides a calming environment that helps alleviate mental fatigue and encourages relaxation.

Progressive Muscle Relaxation (PMR):

Practicing Progressive Muscle Relaxation involves systematically tensing and then relaxing different muscle groups. This technique promotes physical relaxation, reducing muscle tension and overall stress levels.

Volunteer Work and Community Engagement:

Engaging in volunteer work or community activities brings a sense of purpose and connection. Making a positive impact in the community contributes to a more fulfilling life, acting as a buffer against the effects of stress.

Aromatherapy and Essential Oils:

Aromatherapy, using essential oils with calming scents such as lavender or chamomile, can positively impact stress levels. Incorporating these scents into daily routines or using them during relaxation practices offers a sensory approach to stress management.

Laughter Therapy:

Laughter is a natural stress reliever. Engaging in activities that induce laughter, like watching comedy, attending laughter yoga sessions, or spending time with humorous friends, promotes a light-hearted approach to stress management.

Regular Physical Exercise:

Regular physical exercise, whether through aerobic activities, strength training, or sports, releases endorphins — natural mood lifters. Exercise serves as a potent stress reducer, promoting overall well-being.

Technology-Assisted Stress Management Apps:

Using mobile apps designed for stress management provides convenient tools and techniques. These apps often include guided meditations, relaxation exercises, and stress tracking features, offering personalized support.

Breath Control Techniques:

Various breath control techniques, like diaphragmatic breathing or box breathing, offer immediate relief from stress. Incorporating these practices into daily routines enhances overall emotional resilience.

Dedicated Time for Relaxation:

Allocating specific times for relaxation, whether through short breaks during the day or longer sessions on weekends, reinforces a commitment to stress management. Consistent relaxation practices contribute to sustained emotional well-being.

Educational Stress Management Workshops:

Attending stress management workshops provides ongoing education and skill development. These workshops often offer new strategies and insights, empowering individuals to refine their stress management techniques.

Maintaining Healthy Boundaries:

Establishing and maintaining healthy boundaries between personal and professional life is crucial for stress management. Clearly defining priorities and setting realistic expectations contribute to a more balanced lifestyle.

Social Support for Stress Coping:

Talking about stressors with trusted friends, family members, or support groups fosters a sense of connection. Verbalizing concerns and receiving empathetic understanding can significantly alleviate the burden of stress.

Regular Sleep Hygiene Practices:

Prioritizing good sleep hygiene practices, including a consistent sleep schedule and creating a conducive sleep environment, directly influences stress resilience. Quality sleep is fundamental for overall emotional well-being.

Efficiently managing stress involves a combination of mindfulness practices, therapeutic approaches, lifestyle adjustments, and holistic techniques. Tailoring these strategies to individual preferences and integrating them into daily routines contributes to a comprehensive and sustainable stress management plan.

9

Resources and Additional Support

Useful Tools and Apps

Apps for Analysing Blood Sugar Trends:

Examples include Sugar Sense, which delivers intricate insights into patterns and fluctuations, aiding both individuals and healthcare professionals in identifying potential triggers or areas for enhancement in diabetes management.

Apps with Barcode Scanning for Food:

Examples encompass apps like MyFitnessPal, equipped with barcode scanning capabilities to simplify the process of obtaining nutritional information. By scanning product barcodes, users can swiftly access comprehensive information about the food's composition, assisting in making well-informed dietary choices.

Customized Fitness Applications:

Examples include fitness applications such as Nike Training Club, offering customized exercise plans that cater to individual preferences, fitness levels, and health objectives. These applications guide users through workouts, monitor progress, and provide motivation, promoting a consistent and enjoyable fitness routine.

Applications for Tracking Symptoms:

Examples cover apps like mySugr, enabling individuals to log and monitor various diabetes-related symptoms. Maintaining a symptom journal allows users to furnish healthcare professionals with detailed information during consultations, facilitating more precise assessments.

Apps Reminding for Water Intake:

Examples, like WaterMinder, encourage individuals to stay adequately hydrated by sending notifications to prompt regular water consumption throughout the day.

Apps for Diabetes-Friendly Travel Planning:

Examples, such as Diabetes M, provide information on diabetes-friendly restaurants, local medical facilities, and travel tips, aiding in planning and navigating trips while effectively managing diabetes.

Calculators for Insulin Doses:

Examples like RapidCalc assist individuals in determining accurate insulin doses based on factors such as blood glucose levels, carbohydrate intake, and correction factors, contributing to precise and personalized insulin management.

Virtual Grocery Shopping Applications:

Examples, like Instacart, offer convenience by enabling online grocery orders for individuals with diabetes. Some apps may also suggest diabetes-friendly products and provide nutritional information for informed choices.

Emergency Information Apps:

Examples, such as ICE Medical Standard, store vital health details, such as medical conditions, medications, and emergency contacts, ensuring that critical information is readily accessible in case of a health emergency.

Applications for Modifying Recipes:

Examples include apps like Eat This Much, assisting individuals in making diabetes-friendly adjustments to their preferred recipes by proposing alternative ingredients, portion sizes, and cooking methods.

Connectivity Apps for Blood Glucose Meters:

Examples such as One Drop facilitate the smooth transfer of blood sugar readings to a digital platform, enhancing the ability to track and analyse blood glucose trends over time.

Apps for Peer-Reviewed Health Research:

Examples like PubMed Mobile allow individuals to stay informed about the latest advancements in diabetes research by providing access to summaries, key findings, and full-text articles.

Mind-Body Wellness Applications:

Examples, including Headspace, focus on the integration of mental and physical health, offering features such as guided meditation, stress reduction exercises, and holistic well-being practices.

Community Challenges and Competitions Apps:

Examples like Strava organize community challenges or competitions, encouraging individuals to set and achieve health-related goals collectively, fostering a sense of camaraderie and motivation within the community.

Meal Subscription Services Applications:

Examples, such as Freshly, with dedicated apps offer a convenient way for individuals to access diabetes-friendly meal options, providing pre-portioned and nutritionally balanced meals tailored to specific dietary needs.

Continuous Glucose Monitoring (CGM) Apps:

Examples associated with continuous glucose monitoring systems, like Dexcom G6, provide real-time insights into blood glucose levels, allowing users to track trends, set alerts, and make informed decisions about their diabetes management based on continuous data.

Personal Health Record (PHR) Apps:

Examples such as Apple Health serve as centralized repositories for health-related information, allowing users to store medical history, test results, and other relevant data, enhancing communication with healthcare providers and ensuring comprehensive care.

Financial Assistance and Insurance Applications:

Examples, including GoodRx, provide information on financial assistance programs and insurance coverage, supporting individuals in navigating the financial aspects of diabetes management and offering guidance on accessing affordable medications and healthcare services.

Educational Games for Diabetes Learning:

Examples like Dario engage users through interactive and gamified experiences, making learning about diabetes enjoyable and accessible, especially for younger individuals or those who prefer a more interactive approach.

Medication Cost Comparison Applications:

Examples, such as Blink Health, help individuals find affordable options for diabetes medications by providing information on prices, discounts, and generic alternatives, assisting users in making cost-effective choices.

Apps for Meal Timing and Reminders:

Examples like Mealime with meal timing and reminders functionalities assist individuals in maintaining consistent eating schedules, contributing to better blood sugar control and overall adherence to meal plans.

Glucometer Calibration Applications:

Examples of apps that assist in glucometer calibration, like BG Monitor Diabetes, ensure the accuracy of blood glucose readings by guiding users through the calibration process, contributing to reliable monitoring and management.

These examples represent a diverse array of apps available for different purposes in diabetes management. It's important to explore and choose apps that align with individual preferences, needs, and device compatibility. Additionally, app availability may vary based on geographical location and platform (iOS or Android).

Online Communities and Support Groups (Expanded)

Digital communities and online support groups play a crucial role in connecting individuals with diabetes, offering a platform for shared experiences, information exchange, and emotional support. ***Exploring these virtual spaces reveals various advantages and dynamics that contribute to the well-being of participants:***

1. Peer Support:

Online support groups create connections among individuals sharing similar diabetes experiences, fostering emotional understanding and mitigating feelings of isolation.

2. Knowledge Sharing:

These groups facilitate the sharing of practical tips, personal strategies, and up-to-date information on diabetes management, empowering members with valuable insights.

3. Emotional Well-Being:

Recognizing the emotional challenges of diabetes, these virtual communities provide a safe outlet for expressing feelings and sharing coping strategies, positively impacting mental well-being.

4. Motivation and Encouragement:

Celebrating successes, whether big or small, within these groups creates a positive environment that motivates individuals to remain dedicated to their diabetes management goals.

5. Real-Time Q&A:

Participants can seek real-time advice and solutions from the community, enabling effective troubleshooting and sharing of experiences to address specific challenges.

6. Diversity in Perspectives:

Online groups bring together individuals with diverse backgrounds and lifestyles, enriching discussions and providing a broad range of insights into managing diabetes in various contexts.

7. Advocacy and Awareness:

Some groups engage in advocacy, raising awareness about diabetes-related issues, promoting education, and contributing to broader efforts to improve diabetes care.

8. Expert Involvement:

Organizing sessions with healthcare professionals or experts in diabetes management allows members to receive expert advice and evidence-based information.

9. Online Events and Challenges:

Group-organized online events and challenges enhance interaction among members, fostering a sense of community and engagement.

10. Community Guidelines and Moderation:

Effective online support groups establish clear guidelines and moderation to maintain a safe and respectful environment, free from harmful misinformation.

11. Localized Connections:

Some groups facilitate connections based on geographical location, leading to localized support networks and friendships.

12. Crisis Support and Emergency Resources:

In critical situations, online support groups serve as sources of immediate assistance, sharing emergency resources and guidance for urgent scenarios.

13.Interactive Platforms:

Utilizing multimedia elements such as webinars, live chats, and forums enhances the dynamism of discussions and accommodates diverse communication preferences.

14.Positive Reinforcement and Hope:

Sharing success stories and positive experiences within the community instils hope and optimism, motivating those facing challenges in their diabetes journey.

15.Continuous Learning Opportunities: Community-organized webinars and live streams offer continuous learning, featuring expert speakers and educational content to support ongoing knowledge development.

16.Mental Health Support Networks: Specific groups focus on the intersection of diabetes and mental health, providing resources and discussions to address the emotional aspects of living with diabetes.

17.Gender-Specific Diabetes Communities: Communities addressing gender-specific considerations provide open spaces for discussions on unique challenges faced by individuals of different genders.

18.Collaboration with Advocacy Organizations:

Engaging with diabetes advocacy organizations allows members to participate in collective efforts, contribute to awareness campaigns, and join policy discussions related to diabetes.

Online support groups and communities, with their diverse benefits, significantly contribute to the holistic well-being of individuals with diabetes. These digital spaces not only offer information and emotional support but also create a sense of community and collective

empowerment.

Conclusion

To conclude, successfully navigating Type 2 diabetes demands a thorough understanding of the condition and practical strategies for effective management. Throughout this guide, I've explored critical aspects crucial for those recently diagnosed with diabetes. Let's recap the essential points and conclude with an optimistic outlook for a healthier future.

Recap of Key Points:
Understanding Type 2 Diabetes:

I examined the fundamentals of Type 2 diabetes, shedding light on its origins, symptoms, and the importance of early identification.

Effects on the Body:

Discussing the impact on the body, I stressed the importance of awareness and proactive measures to minimize complications.

Lifestyle Adjustments:

Lifestyle changes emerged as pivotal, highlighting the role of diet, exercise, and habits in diabetes management.

Nutritional Requirements:

The section on meal planning fundamentals clarified the nutritional needs for diabetics, emphasizing balanced, mindful eating.

Portion Control and Food Choices:

Recognizing the significance of portion control and selecting appropriate foods, I highlighted practical approaches to foster healthier dietary habits.

Diabetic-Friendly Recipes:

Exploring various meal options, I presented recipes for breakfast, lunch, dinner, and snacks tailored to meet nutritional goals.

Weekly Meal Plans:

I explored crafting sample meal plans for diverse preferences, focusing on nutrient balance throughout the week.

Managing Blood Sugar Levels:

Strategies for monitoring and testing, adjusting meal plans, and integrating physical activity were emphasized as crucial components of effective blood sugar management.

Tips for Dining Out:

Insightful tips for making healthy choices at restaurants and navigating social situations provided practical guidance for maintaining dietary goals away from home.

Emotional Well-Being:

Coping with the diagnosis, building support systems, and managing stress were discussed to address the emotional aspects of living with diabetes.

Resources and Additional Support:

I highlighted the abundance of resources, including useful tools and apps, and the value of community and online support groups for comprehensive diabetes management.

Embarking on the journey of managing Type 2 diabetes, recognize that every step toward a healthier lifestyle propels you toward a brighter future. Consistency in adopting the principles discussed—whether in nutrition, physical activity, or emotional well-being—holds the key to effective diabetes management.

Take pride in your progress, and don't hesitate to seek support from healthcare professionals, online communities, and available resources. Diabetes management is an evolving process, and your commitment to self-care lays the foundation for a healthier and more fulfilling life.

View challenges as opportunities for growth and adaptation. With informed choices, a positive mindset, and the support of those around you, managing Type 2 diabetes becomes an empowering journey towards sustained well-being.

May your path be marked with resilience, positive transformations, and a commitment to nurturing your health. Here's to a future filled with vitality, well-being, and the triumphs that come with a balanced and mindful approach to life with Type 2 diabetes.

9 7 9 8 8 7 7 7 2 2 1 3 2